Back Care for Carers

by Andrew Bellamy

Illustrations by Pat Glentworth

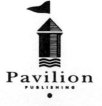

Pavilion
PUBLISHING

BACK CARE FOR CARERS

A self-help guide for carers on prevention and management of back pain

Published by Pavilion Publishing (Brighton) Ltd.
8 St George's Place,
Brighton,
East Sussex BN1 4GB
Telephone: 01273 623222
Fax: 01273 625526

© Andrew Bellamy, 1995.

Illustrations © Pat Glentworth, 1995.

First published 1995.

ISBN 1 871080 44 4

A catalogue record for this book is available from the British Library.

Editor: Anna McGrail
Design & typesetting: Stanford Douglas
Printed by: Page Bros (Norwich)

Carers have a Duty of Care

The term may be incompatible with itself, but I am advocating a little *selfish altruism*; take the Duty of Care as an important principle and apply it to yourself as well as to those for whom you care. By their very nature, carers tend to look after others and neglect themselves. This is noble but counter-productive. Your healthy body is your essential equipment. Neglect it, and you, your work and your patient will suffer.

To Mum

Contents

The Author

Andrew Bellamy is an osteopath who works full-time in his own practice dealing with a wide range of conditions affecting the musculo-skeletal system. Much of his work involves injuries to the lower back although he has a special interest in the management of chronic disease.

Andrew initially trained as a State Registered Nurse, specialising in operating theatre work; this stimulated his interest in human anatomy and the way it functions. It also initiated a wish to try to work in an holistic manner, aiming at the prevention of injury and the maintenance of health as well as corrective and remedial methods.

He undertook a five-year course at the London School of Osteopathy, graduating in 1988, where he is now a Member of Faculty, teaching Applied Osteopathy. In addition, Andrew is a council member of the Natural Therapeutic and Osteopathic Society and Register.

Experience gained within the NHS has helped in establishing good relations with local medical professionals. Andrew works with his father, a retired General Practitioner and qualified osteopath. Much of his time with patients is spent instructing them in preventative techniques and exercises.

Foreword

It is a great privilege to have been asked to write the foreword to Andrew's book. Andrew is a well known and respected osteopath who gives his all to his patients. It is this desire to help which has motivated him to write this guide: to try to prevent people from injuring themselves.

The emphasis throughout on the prevention of problems is tremendous. Only later does he go on to deal with the treatment of problems after they have occurred.

The book is set out sensibly, in an easy-to-read format, and in such a way that you can quickly brush up on a specific exercise or find help with a particular problem.

I feel that this is an excellent reference book for all carers and recommend it whole-heartedly.

Dr Tim Stevenson

MB, BCH, BAO, DRCOG, MRCGP

General Practitioner

Acknowledgements

Thank you to Pat and our children who put up with me ignoring them while I completed this, to my father for his encouragement, assistance and contribution, and to my patients who have given me food for thought. Special thanks to Mary Colato, of the East Sussex Carers, Bridie Asquith of Southlands Hospital Occupational Health Department and Mike Morris, DO.

Introduction

The subject of back care is important to us all.

Almost everyone will experience some form of musculo-skeletal injury during their lives. For most of us, this means an uncomfortable and relatively short period during which we can expect the sympathy and attention of others as we recover.

Yet one group in our society, whether professionals or volunteers, has to face the consequences of injury on a daily basis. These are the carers amongst us.

For carers, an understanding of good lifting technique and how to avoid and manage back injuries has a direct effect upon the safety and comfort of others. This book is aimed at both the professional carers, such as nurses and care-assistants, and those who rightly consider themselves 'professional' even though they do not receive a salary for the care that they give. Carers who have to look after a child with disabilities, an elderly relative, friend or spouse who has had a stroke, often have to do so 24 hours a day.

This book has two main areas of emphasis. The **avoidance** of injury is a major priority for all carers and so advice on this is an important part of the text. However, it has to be recognised that injuries do occur and so the other main focus of the book is upon **self-help** and the subsequent prevention of further problems. I hope that while you read this book you will keep in mind the principle that prevention really is better than cure

Whilst we all have a responsibility for those around us, carers have a **Duty of Care**. I judge this to mean that carers have a duty to care for themselves as well for their charges.

Inevitably, the subject of back care is a vast one that cannot be covered fully in this text. However, I hope that readers will be able to gain a basic understanding of anatomy, how injuries occur and what they can do to avoid an injured back, as well as how to help themselves if they do suffer an injury.

Osteopathy and Carers

Osteopathy is probably the best known of the complementary health professions; about one million people visit osteopaths every year in the United Kingdom alone. This gives practitioners an enviable experience in diagnosing and managing mechanical problems involving the muscles and joints of the body.

Even if one sees osteopaths simply as 'spinal mechanics', they are in a privileged position to give you good advice about your back and, if necessary, treat any problems that arise.

There is more to it than manipulation of the spine. Osteopaths believe that structural problems of the musculo-skeletal system can affect the whole of one's well being. A simple toothache can make us feel rotten, so why are we so surprised when we are not at our best when we have backache?

Osteopaths, as holistic practitioners, aim to treat the musculo-skeletal system so that the whole person can achieve a healthy state. If you give it the opportunity, the body will try to help itself. We call this **homeostasis**, a term familiar to every medical person. In practical terms, this means that the body will use its inherent ability to heal itself, as long as we remove the obstacles to healing. Osteopaths express this in the aphorism 'structure governs function'.

So the modern, well-trained osteopath is more than a bone-setter. While it is true that some problems are resolved with 'one quick snap', most of our work is less dramatic than that. Direct manual therapy is, of course, very important. However, all good osteopaths also act as advisors on posture, exercise and the management of injuries. In addition, they are trained to recognise other patterns of illness and disability. They are able to liaise well with other health professionals, and to direct the patient to the most appropriate specialist, whether general practitioner, surgeon, physiotherapist, chiropodist, acupuncturist or other therapist.

Some patients are reluctant to approach their general practitioner initially, but have been helped when the osteopath has discovered diabetes or high blood pressure and referred them appropriately.

On a more personal level, the osteopath has the time to listen and provide a foil for the many concerns and stresses that people face today. These stresses contribute considerably to the natural history of many people's problems, and a listening ear can help to remove some of the obstacles to getting back to full health.

By their very nature, carers tend to look after others and neglect themselves. However noble this may be, it tends to be counter-productive. As a carer, your healthy body is your essential equipment; if you neglect it, you, your work and your patient will suffer. I believe that this is a good enough reason to adopt the osteopathic way of thinking.

Remember these three basic osteopathic principles:

- The human body, starting out healthy, will maintain its own health if given the opportunity.

- Every part of you influences all of you, body and psyche.

- The way that your body is constructed governs the way it works and vice versa.

Try to adopt an osteopathic way of thinking, looking at the way that you do things, at home and at work. Use the stretches and exercises in this book, use them sensibly and regularly. Think in terms of preventing musculo-skeletal injuries rather than treating them after they have arisen.

Anatomy and Physiology

If you have some understanding of how your spine is constructed, how it works and what can go wrong if it is badly looked after, you will be better placed to understand the relevance of the advice and exercises in this book. Please take a few minutes to study this section so that you have some understanding of your own back. Additionally, you may be able to advise others on why prevention of injury is so important and therefore extend your role as a carer.

The spinal column

The human spine is made up of bones called vertebrae, their joints, muscles, ligaments, blood vessels, the spinal cord and its nerves. All these are ultimately covered by skin, and every one of these components (and many others) can be a source of back pain. Some back pains come from irritation or compression of the nerves that leave the spine and go to all parts of your body. Its purpose is to support us in an upright and balanced way that allows walking and the many movements that we make throughout our lives.

Many factors affect the ability of the spine to work effectively and, for many of us, injuries and poor posture or working conditions only add to the normal changes that occur with ageing. Misuse, abuse or accident can lead to loss of function and to pain.

The vertebrae

The vertebrae are divided into several groups; the neck, (seven cervical vertebrae), the mid-back, (twelve dorsal vertebrae), the lower back, (five lumbar vertebrae), the sacrum and the tail bone (coccyx).

A typical vertebra is made up of three main parts: a body, which lies in front, an arch formed by two 'spines' or processes that project sideways and one which projects backwards, and two pairs of joints that link one vertebra to its neighbours above and below.

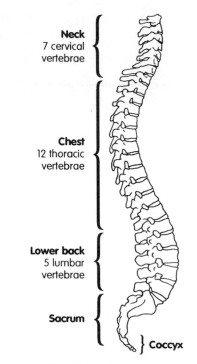

Neck
7 cervical vertebrae

Chest
12 thoracic vertebrae

Lower back
5 lumbar vertebrae

Sacrum

} **Coccyx**

The spinal column

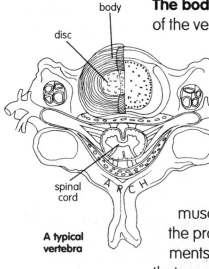

disc

body

spinal cord

A R C H

A typical vertebra

The body provides much of the weight-bearing ability of the vertebrae, which are separated from one another by the inter-vertebral discs. It has a relatively large surface area.

The arch contains and protects the spinal cord and its nerves. The portion of the arch that projects backwards is the part that one can feel under the skin. This, together with another pair of processes that project sideways, provides anchor points for muscles and ligaments. Muscles that pass between the processes allow the wide range of spinal move-ments that are possible, as well as the spinal bracing that we need for normal balance.

Above and below the arch are two pairs of **facet joints**. These link and stabilise the vertebrae and guide the movement that takes place between each neighbouring vertebra. Generally the facet joints allow forward and backwards motion but limit sideways motion. They are surrounded by a sac or capsule, the lining of which produces a slick, low-friction synovial fluid that helps the joints to glide easily.

When the spine is bent forward, the joints separate slightly, allowing more sideways and twisting motion. It is at this time that the joints are at their most vulnerable to injury.

The inter-vertebral discs

Between all the vertebrae, except at the sacrum and coccyx, is an inter-vertebral disc. These discs vary in size and thickness depending on which part of the spine they lie in. Those in the lumbar spine are the thickest and widest, demonstrating that these discs take the greatest load. The discs act as shock absorbers, transmitting and spreading much of the force passing through your body.

Discs are made of two main parts, a tough outer fibrous part that is layered for strength and is slightly elastic. Within this, there is a soft, jelly-like inner called the *nucleus pulposus* that provides a degree of 'bounce'. During daily activity, pressure through the spine and discs forces some of the fluids within the nucleus pulposus out. This probably takes place through small channels into the vertebrae above and below.

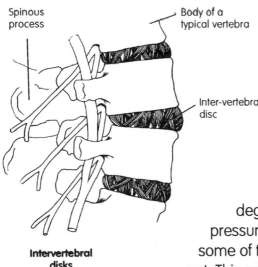

Spinous process

Body of a typical vertebra

Inter-vertebral disc

Intervertebral disks

These fluids are then replaced by diffusion via the same route during rest periods, so that a normal pressure is restored.

The discs mainly allow movement forwards and backwards like a rocking chair, whilst a small amount of sideways movement and shear is possible. As we age, or after injuries, these discs become less elastic, are less able to take in fluids, and tend to thin. The direct result of this is that our spines become generally less flexible.

The nerves

One further important factor in understanding back pain is the nerves that leave the spine to go to the rest of the body. A pair of nerves leaves the spinal cord between each pair of vertebrae through a notch or canal created by the arches of two adjacent vertebrae.

The inter-vertebral disc lies in front of the spinal cord. The cord sits in a canal that goes from the top to the bottom of the spine, and forms part of the central nervous system. The nerves are also initially contained in this canal. Any abnormal pressure onto the cord, at any level of the spine, will interfere with the normal working of the adjacent areas, and also the muscles and organs that are served by those nerves. If there is pressure onto an individual nerve root, then the effects are felt in the parts of the body to which that nerve goes. Symptoms may include pain, numbness or tingling and may be either right- or left-sided. Pressure onto those nerve roots, in the lower back, that form the sciatic nerve cause the leg pains that we call sciatica.

The ligaments

The spine is reinforced by vertebral ligaments that run from the top to the bottom. Two, in particular, provide great stability and control. There is one at the front of the vertebral bodies (anterior longitudinal ligament) and one at the back (posterior longitudinal ligament).

spinal cord

anterior longtitudinal ligament

spinal nerves

posterior longtitudinal ligament

At each level, the discs are encased by these and other ligaments, which support them rather like a corset and yet do not affect their naturally elastic properties. The posterior ligament starts to thin in the lumbar vertebrae as it comes down the spine, until it is only half its original width when it meets the sacrum. Unfortunately, the region where the ligament is at its weakest is also the part of the spine that takes the greatest strain. This is one of the reasons why we suffer most back strains and injuries in the low back.

The trunk muscles

The human body has some 400 muscles, many of which play an important part in good posture. Many of the largest of these muscles are in the trunk of the body, where they control the spine and abdomen and it is therefore most important that they are kept healthy and in good condition.

The stretches and exercises that I recommend in this book are aimed at these areas so that the load upon the spine is minimised.

Maintaining a Healthy Back

In order to maintain your back in a healthy state, you have to be essentially sound in the first place. The term 'maintenance' can be viewed in at least two ways:

● keeping the *status quo* of an already healthy back;

● maintaining restored health after an injury has healed.

Some of the factors that can disturb this principle include: deformity, disease, obesity, pregnancy and poor posture.

Mechanical effects

When I consult a new patient, I like to start with the feet and ankles. The individual may well have a simple, uncomplicated low-back injury, but so often I see mechanical problems in the feet and ankles that may have contributed to the cause of that injury

Bunions　　Commonly, bunions will deform the great toes, causing the feet to turn out slightly and the ankles to lean inwards. The arches of the feet tend to flatten, also altering the normal foot suspension.

The knees often lean inwards also, to help compensate, and this all ultimately leads to adaptations in the pelvis and the lower back. Such patients frequently have an excessive lumbar curve which puts stress on the spine.

Leg length   Differences in leg length can occur as a result of congenital or traumatic events, such as fractures. If one leg is shorter than the other, then the pelvis tilts, forming an uneven and potentially unstable platform for the lumbar spine. If the difference in leg length is more than 1cm (one third of an inch), the mechanical stress upon the pelvis and spine leads to adaptations in posture that alter the normal spinal curves. The tendency is to introduce a scoliosis, or twisting of the spinal column. Muscles, discs, ligaments and tendons have to change their natural length and this disrupts normal balance and affects the body's homeostasis.

Arthritis

Osteo-arthritis or rheumatoid arthritis that affects any of the leg joints or lumbar spine will have an effect upon posture. The joints can become distorted and painful, making normal posture very awkward.

Osteo-arthritis is the type of arthritis that is commonly described as 'wear-and-tear'. The causes are not entirely clear, but age, obesity and joint injury all have a part to play. It is more common in women and symptoms are most likely to appear after the menopause, although I must stress that the link between the two may simply be the age of the patient. The main symptom is pain in the joints which makes itself felt slowly over a period of time. It tends to be most noticeable after exercise.

The causes of rheumatoid arthritis are sadly not fully understood either, but onset of the condition has been linked to severe physical or emotional stress. Most of us would recognise this often crippling disease by the gnarled, painful appearance of a sufferer's finger joints. The disease itself is thought to be one of the auto-immune diseases, where the body's immune system attacks the linings of affected joints. It is twice as common in women than in men and affects about one per cent of the population as a whole.

Obesity

Obesity tilts the pelvis forward because of the weight of the belly, which increases the lumbar curve. Adverse pressure on the lumbar discs and ligaments makes it difficult for an obese person to maintain a correct posture. Ultimately it becomes too late to make a full return to normal.

The same effect can come from high-heeled shoes; if worn habitually, they throw body weight forward onto the great-toe joints. Bunions and fallen arches are a frequent feature in obesity and may be partly due to this excessive pressure.

Pregnancy

Pregnancy has a similar effect on the body to obesity but is, of course, short-term. It is vital, however, after a pregnancy, that extra care is taken to get posture back to normal, especially as this is a time when women are usually thinking less about their own health and more about their new responsibilities.

Posture

This is a crucial area on which to focus when considering our general body health and particularly that of the spine. It is also a subject on which there is contrasting opinion. One thing that most people seem to agree upon is that

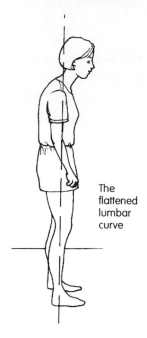

The flattened lumbar curve

poor posture frequently leads to back problems. General postural faults such as slouching and sitting poorly will ultimately cause back pain. Your mother was quite right when she told you to sit up straight. People with poor posture often have flattened or reduced lumbar curves. However, the military-type posture is just as undesirable because it forces the spine to straighten the natural curves.

Remember: the fact that you do not suffer from back problems does not automatically mean that you have good posture.

Postural Tips

Do:	Don't:
Think tall	Play down your height if you are tall.
Stand with knees loose.	'Lock' out your knees.
Keep your back and stomach muscles strong.	Avoid exercise.
Concentrate on keeping your head position level.	Let yourself get overweight.
Keep your eyes ahead rather than down or up.	Let bunions or flat feet develop.
Adopt a good head and neck position; this makes the rest much easier.	Wear high-heeled shoes regularly.
Use a chair with good lumbar and thigh support, especially at work.	Slouch in chairs, at home or at work.
Take regular breaks when driving any distance.	Move your driving mirror; sit up instead.
Straighten up and stretch after bending.	

Remember: a stooped posture in old age is not inevitable. Of course disease and such factors as osteoporosis have an effect, but let's not submit to them just because we are getting older. If you keep fit, eat healthily and maintain good posture, postural changes can be delayed and you may even prevent some of the problems of old age.

Checking your own posture

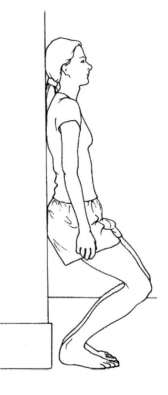

- Stand with your back to a wall in a posture normal for you, heels four centimetres, (two inches), away from it.

- Rest so that calves, buttocks and shoulder blades are touching the wall. (Most people's heads do not touch).

- Slide down the wall by bending your knees until your head does touch the wall.

- Keep relaxed and stand up, keeping your head touching the wall.

- Walk away from the wall; this should be your correct posture.

At the start your new posture may feel awkward and even uncomfortable. You may be changing decades of bad habits, so keep practising!

Alexander Technique

Many people are now attending classes in Alexander Technique. It teaches you what postural mistakes you are making and how to train yourself to avoid them. For those who need the discipline of instruction, I would recommend looking for a class.

General considerations in handling

Much research has been undertaken on the risks to people while they handle loads, whether the loads are other people or inanimate objects. Assessing the risks and implementing ways to reduce them might be considered a shorthand definition for the term **ergonomics**.

For many, the phrase 'an ergonomic design' conjures up an image of a strangely shaped Swedish chair, or cutlery for the elderly arthritic. Ergonomics goes further than this, however, and looks at the relationship between us and our surroundings, attempting — as far as is possible — to fit the job to the employee and not the other way around.

One simple example of ergonomics is that of a foot-rail in a pub. If, at the end of a long day, you stand with one foot on the rail, you brace the opposite knee and hip, relieving stress on the lower back. This makes you more comfortable and so encourages you to stay longer.

When we are comfortable doing our job, injuries are much less likely, stress and resentment do not build up and, most importantly, the person for whom you are caring is much better cared for.

The assessment of risk for any task lies ultimately with you, your employer, or both of you. Whether or not you are paid to care, there is a duty to remove or reduce risk as far as possible. Tasks that have always been done manually in the past may not need to be. The attitude of 'Well, we've always done it that way' simply is not good enough. I would like to suggest that every carer also has a responsibility to think about the specific tasks he or she is doing, and ask for changes if there is a workable alternative.

Even if the main responsibility for care and safety falls to someone else, please do not wait until someone is injured and then say, 'We've always said that was going to happen one day.'

For many carers, their responsibilities inevitably take them outside the employer's direct control. Often your place of work is in someone else's home, so try to get into the habit of making your own assessment of the risks that you face. Those of you who are employed carers need to remember that much of the training and advice that your employer will give will be of a general nature.

Those who care *without* specific training face additional risks. Listed below are some of the factors that you might like to think about as part of judging what risks you and your patient face.

Look carefully at what you do. Ask what it involves, and do this *before* you start.

- Do you have to support your patient away from your body?

- Are you twisting your trunk? Can you avoid this?

- Is your posture such that you are stooping or over-reaching? Can you avoid this?

- Are you moving or lifting the patient further than you need to? Can you reduce the distance?

- Are you pulling or pushing; for example, dragging a chair with someone still in it? Can this be avoided?

- Finally, very importantly for many carers, how long have you already been working? Should you be taking a break?

Some estimates suggest that nursing staff spend as much as 30% of their working day in a stooped position.*

All of the following are common-sense pieces of advice, but it's surprising how often, especially when we are rushed, tired and have many demands put on us, we can push them to one side for the sake of short-term expediency.

*Health and Safety Commission (1992): *Guidance on Manual Handling of Loads in the Health Services.*

● With specific regard to your lower back, tasks such as bathing a patient, dressing them, changing dressings for leg ulcers or other wounds, require a lot of bending down. Where possible, kneel rather than crouch; not only is it kinder to your back, but you are more likely to be properly stable for the job you have to do.

● Arrange the things you need like dressing packs or toiletries within easy reach, particularly in such a position that avoids you having to twist.

● The sort of position that involves being bent forward and then twisting to one side is typical of the reported history of patients suffering with acute lower-back strain. **Avoid it.**

Ways to Lift

The way in which we lift or move a patient is very important both to the lifter and the lifted. People are not a convenient shape to handle, and sometimes cannot or will not always co-operate easily. It is crucial that the person to be moved and the 'mover' work together so that the load is spread as evenly as possible.

Perhaps the commonest lifts or moves are from one seated position to another, involving beds, commodes and armchairs. The basic principles of good lifting technique will apply to most combinations and can be adapted to suit individual circumstances. Much also depends on the ability of the patient to help themselves; it may therefore be necessary to teach patients the technique and the importance of working in unison.

When we watch toddlers lifting something, we see that they usually do the following:

- They stand directly in front of and slightly over the object.

- They bend both knees but keep their arms straight and slip their hands underneath the object.

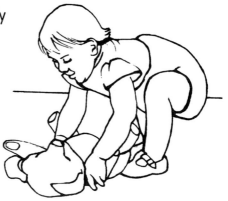

- They usually hold the object close to the body and perform the lift substantially with the legs.

- When letting something to the floor, they will often allow it to slide down the front of their thighs.

This technique is exactly how we should all lift and would appear to be the 'natural' way to do so.

Make sure that you get in the habit of doing the following when you lift:

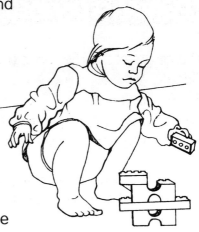

- Do not rush.

- Decide who will give the commands.

- Start your combined movements by rocking gently to create some momentum.

- Don't drag your patient. This will often cause them to pull back and could injure you both.

- Arrange any furniture involved so that the distance between is minimised.

- Move furniture that is not needed out of the way. In a home situation, this can easily be established as a permanent situation, reducing risk.

- Put on wheelchair and bed brakes where appropriate.

- Where possible, keep furniture height even.

- Keep pets out while you are lifting.

Most home lifting involves at most two people: the carer and the cared for. I shall describe techniques that involve these two individuals although I stress that, wherever possible, **two** carers should be involved in any lifting activity. It is regrettable that in too many circumstances the carer is working alone and so the precautions are even more important.

1 TRANSFER HOLD, (BELT TYPE)

The height of the lifter does not matter for this technique. This method of lifting is also very comforting for most patients, as they feel securely 'held'. It is my preference because the lifter has a good grip at a low centre of gravity and is not required to bend too much. With practice, this method of lifting requires very little effort.

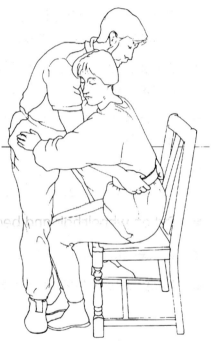

- Stand in front of the patient and slightly to one side.

- Place one foot beside the patient and the other in front of their feet, blocking their knees with your leg.

- Reach under the arms and grasp the patient's belt or waist-band firmly, using the whole hand.

- The patient can now steady themselves and push up from the chair or use your hips for support as they lean forward.

 In patients who have suffered a stroke, there is often one side of the body that is weaker. Not only may one leg or arm be weaker, but the patient may also have less co-ordination. Make sure that you stand and support on the weaker side.

The four lifts described in these pages have been adapted with kind permission from the National Back Pain Association's book *The Guide to the the Handling of Patients.*

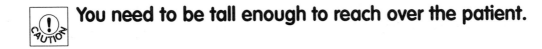

2 TRANSFER HOLD, (ELBOW TYPE)

This simply varies the first hold. Remember that only one person should be giving the instructions!

 You need to be tall enough to reach over the patient.

Where possible, ask the patient to shift to the front of the seat.

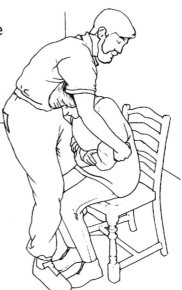

- Stand in front of the patient and slightly to one side.

- Place one foot beside the patient and the other in front of their feet, blocking their knees with your knee and thigh.

- Once you are balanced, ask the patient to lean forward into your body.

- Reach over the patient's back and clasp both elbows, ensuring a firm grip.

- The diagram shows how your arm locks the shoulder that is further from you by coming in front.

- With a co-ordinated effort, the patient can now be assisted on to their feet. Minimum effort for you and maximum stability for the patient.

This lift is most useful where space is minimal and is very useful in helping the patient upright or to move to a new seat.

3 PATIENT-ASSISTED BED LIFT

Where you are alone and have to move a patient onto or further up a bed, first assess the patient's ability to manage themselves. Having decided how much assistance they need, you can then prepare to help.

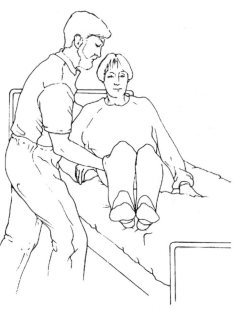

- Where possible, ask the patient to sit on the edge of the bed.

- Ask the patient to shuffle to the head end of the bed in small 'hops'.

- Stand to the side of the patient nearest the head end.

- Bend your knees and support the patient by placing one arm across the shoulders and the other under the thighs.

- Ask the patient to lean back at your command.

- As the patient leans back, lift the patient's thighs and turn towards the bed, while also supporting the upper body.

 Move with the patient so that you remain close. This close contact helps you and also reassures the patient. Avoid twisting and leaning forward.

4 PATIENT-ASSISTED ONE-PERSON LIFT

This hold should only be contemplated when there is no alternative and the patient is light and able to help. If two people are available, this lift can be used with one carer on each side of the patient, using one arm each.

- Seat the patient on the side of the bed and swing them on using the patient-assisted bed lift described above.

- Ask the patient to grasp one of their own wrists with their strongest hand and to hold both the arms close to the body.

- Now ask the patient to bend their strongest leg at the knee in preparation to assist the lift. A secure bolster at the foot of the bed may help to give something to push against.

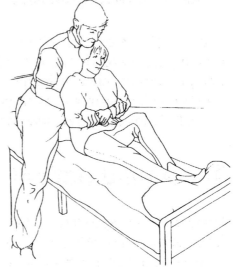

- Kneel behind the patient on the bed. Pass your arms under the patient's armpits and grasp their forearms near to the elbow.

- Keep your arms straight and, on an agreed command, ask the patient to push with the bent leg whilst you lift to the head of the bed.

 Do not let the patient interlock the fingers as this can lead to strains.

 Keep your own back as straight as possible.

Lifting in Special Situations

The spastic patient

Spastic patients can sometimes move their limbs with considerable force and apparently randomly. To minimise this, encourage the patient to start and perform as much of the movement as possible. Always start by rocking, and keep all movements as smooth as possible. Do not straighten the patient's limbs out too rapidly as this can trigger reflex activity.

The young patient

Lifting and moving young children and babies can offer as many opportunities for back injuries as lifting adults can, so the fact that they are relatively light can be deceiving. Children are often low down or behind cot sides, sometimes fractious and unco-operative. A carer often has to move suddenly as children tend to have little conception of danger. When carried, they offer an awkward and mobile package — usually just when you need a hand free to do something else. In short, we take risks with children that we probably would not with an adult patient. If the child has disabilities, the risks are compounded.

Train yourself to do the common-sense things that are listed below:

- Make sure cot sides are down.

- Kneel instead of stooping.

- Try not to squat as not only can this damage your knee cartilages, but you can also be knocked off balance.

- Carry the child close to your body. Support the child from below using one arm, with your other arm around the child's body.

- Avoid carrying on the hip as this can aggravate back conditions.

- Think about any disability the child may have and plan the lift in advance.

When handling a small child, you will have to bend to lift them off the floor, so it is important that the child feels secure. A sense of security helps to prevent a child from struggling, which could threaten your stability.

Lifting a child from the floor

(assuming the child is face down)

- Half kneel beside the child, with one foot flat and with that knee bent.

- Slide one hand under the child's shoulders and gently cradle the far shoulder.

- Pass your other hand between the child's legs and under the abdomen.

- Bracing your legs and keeping a straight back, lift the child towards you, turning them slightly so that the child's back is in firm contact with you.

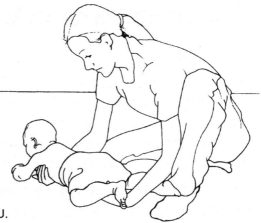

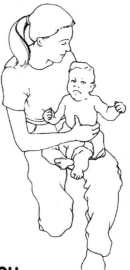

- Bring the child upright and settle him or her onto your thigh and into a seated position.

- Now, with one hand across the child's chest and one supporting beneath the child, you can stand.

 Use the same basic hand-hold when lifting a child from a cot but, as you have to lean slightly, bring the child to the side of the cot before lifting.

 Avoid twisting as you stand. Move your feet so that they point in the direction you want to go.

 Do not be tempted to adjust bedding or pull back covers whilst holding a child. Arrange these before you lift.

The patient who falls

It is probable that all carers will have to deal with a patient who falls. The patient may faint, be epileptic or simply become fatigued and need to rest, choosing you as the support. Some patients can also be difficult or aggressive and falling is a good way to make a point. Both lifter and lifted can be injured. Your duty of care is to ensure that the patient is kept safe but also to make sure that you are fit to help them to their feet or call for assistance if necessary.

It is quite natural to try to stop a patient from falling, but it is far safer to allow the patient to slide to the floor in a controlled way, as described overleaf.

- Be aware of where the patient's weight is in relation to you. If the patient starts to lean heavily on you, be prepared.

- Increase your support, i.e. grasp one of the patient's hands and put your other arm firmly around their waist.

- Use your thigh to support the patient; lean them towards you, not away.

- Ease the patient and yourself down to the floor, either onto their knees or, if necessary, into the recovery position.

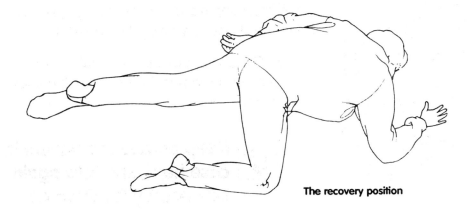

The recovery position

I do not believe that there can be a prescribed way to move a patient into the recovery position as each instance will be different. However, the main principles can always be followed.

- Protect the patient's head at all times.

- Once the patient is on the floor, ensure that he or she is comfortable.

- Make sure that neither of you is injured before attempting to move the patient.

 Practise this manoeuvre before you undertake any role as a carer.

Getting the patient up

Often a patient who has fallen needs only a short time to recover and then you can continue.

If the patient can sit up by themselves, help them first onto their knees and then upright. Use this method:

- Stand behind the patient, supporting their back with your knees and thighs.

- Support the patient by holding them under their armpits and assist them onto their knees by lifting, keeping your arms straight, knees bent and back as straight as possible.

- Once your patient is on their knees, rest for a moment before assisting them to their feet.

Keep behind the patient in case he or she falls again. Use nearby furniture as a prop where possible.

 If the patient cannot help themselves into a sitting position, the reason for their fall may require medical help. If you have to get down to floor level yourself to haul a patient up, not only do you risk personal injury, but the patient is probably not in a fit state to be lifted anyway.

Where there is any doubt, it is important that you make sure the patient is comfortably in the recovery position, that he or she is breathing freely, and that you get assistance.

Maintenance Plan

This plan describes an exercise programme that can be used by carers both to help *prevent* injuries and to help you *recover* after an injury. Whatever your circumstances, this series of exercises will help you to achieve a higher level of fitness and offers some protection against future back problems. I hope that, once you have followed the plan, you will feel inspired to take up some full-time sport or activity that will improve your general health even further. For more information on suitable activities, see the section on **Keeping Healthy** on page 59.

You will find that this maintenance plan relates mainly to the lower back but will identify specific areas where appropriate.

General pointers

- Do your exercises when you have time, but please make sure that you are not rushing simply to get them out of the way.

- Keep a note of how you are progressing.

 Write it down if you want; for example, record where pain is felt, if it moves and to which part of the body. Record how may repetitions of each exercise you do.

- Most exercises suggest a number of repetitions. Don't worry if ten or twenty repetitions are suggested and you can only do five, work up to the suggested number as you improve.

- When you do *any* exercise, breathe **out** when making an effort, **in** when relaxing.

- Study the techniques involved carefully so that you are confident that you know what to do.

- These exercises are intended in part to prevent you from developing injuries, but also help you recover from them and return you to normal. Sometimes this means, therefore, that you may have to stretch or bend a joint or a section of your back until it is uncomfortable.

- If a particular exercise causes sustained pain, you must stop. It may simply mean that you are being too enthusiastic, but it can also suggest that you are not yet ready for that particular exercise.

- Even if you have only been suffering from back pain in one small area, try the exercises that focus on other areas of the body as well. Remember that the back is a single unit, made up of linked parts, not parts on their own.

 If you are not sure what is safe and relevant for you, seek professional advice from an osteopath or chartered physiotherapist. If you do not know of one in your area, addresses of professional bodies can be found under Sources of Further Information on page 111.

 Properly performed exercises will still be of use to you after any pain from an injury has gone. Make your exercises part of your daily routine.

Age and gender

I am often asked whether there is an age limit to both treatment and exercise. Does one's gender matter? In my view, there is no limit as long one adopts an appropriate attitude. I, along with many other osteopaths, treat patients who range from infants to octogenarians... and occasionally beyond. What has to change is the approach. An eighty-year-old woman with osteoporosis must be treated differently to a fifteen-year-old boy who injures a knee falling off a bike. The same applies to exercise and sport: tailor the mode of exercise to the body that needs it.

Precautions

I make no attempt to diagnose from a distance, as all of you have different individual circumstances, levels of fitness and are of different ages. There are a number of points, however, to be considered before attempting any of the exercises.

● Those who are or may be pregnant should always take advice, although this does not mean that you are excluded. For example, those in their first trimester should avoid any stomach-toning exercises, while others can be undertaken if supervised.

● Those with pre-existing conditions or who are receiving medication must check with their general practitioner before beginning an exercise programme.

Stretching and warming up before exercise

Always make sure that you follow a stretching and warm-up routine before you do any exercise. For all sports, you need to stretch and warm up in a slow and progressive manner. Particularly after vigorous exercise, warm down as well. The process varies with individual sports, as described below.

While stretching and warming up are most important as the precursors to exercise, there is every reason to use the same techniques as a way of improving your everyday suppleness. Remember the importance of injury prevention and the maintenance of good health to you holistically.

For example, for general lower-back toning, you may wish to perform **Exercises 6 (Knee to chest)**, **7 (Pelvic tilting)** and **8 (Roll-up)**, as a way of loosening up first thing in the morning. These can be done every day and they can all be performed before you even leave your bed!

Try all of the suggested exercises and keep a note of those that were easy and those that were less so. Concentrate on the less easy ones, build up slowly the number of repetitions and the number of times you do them. Try the exercises once or twice every day to start with and you will soon find the level that keeps you, as an individual, more supple. Some people will need to continue with daily stretches, others perhaps two to three times per week.

When using these techniques for sports preparation, even those who exercise regularly tend to stretch for only a couple of minutes. Before jogging or running, for example, you should warm-up for eight to ten minutes. Do not be put off by feeling that you look foolish. You are protecting yourself from the injuries that become almost inevitable as you age and want to continue in sport.

Stretching and warming up (and down) become more and more relevant as you get older, as muscles tend to shorten naturally and you lose many of those fibres that give you muscle bulk and fast response.

One distinction between stretching and warming up is to think of the **stretch** as preparing the body generally and the **warm up** as preparing muscles specific to your activity.

The process of stretching and warming prepares your body by:

- raising the heart rate gently, preparing your cardio-vascular system;

- filling the muscles with well-oxygenated blood;

- helping to make muscles and tendons more flexible and therefore more injury-resistant;

- reducing muscle and joint tension, giving you a greater range of motion;

- improving proprioception, the body's sense of where it is in time and space;

- prepares you mentally for what you are about to do.*

Everyone can stretch. Age or current fitness are not a bar. You simply have to use common sense and follow some simple rules. If you are unsure, check with a professional advisor.

- Stretching must be done slowly.

- You are likely to feel different on different days — take this into account.

- General stretches are best done at the start of the day.

- Avoid bouncing or using powerful, jerky movements.

- Hold the stretch for about 20 seconds to make it effective.

- Do not allow any stretch to be painful.

- Stretch and warm up for eight to ten minutes, longer if you are preparing for vigorous activity, such as jogging.

- Try to stretch specific muscle groups if you will be using them in a particular activity or sport.

If you are naturally stiff, be more careful, but for you stretching is even more important!

Note: Some people will never be able to touch their toes, however hard they practise. So what? You should be bending your knees anyway!

*After Bob Anderson (1981): *Stretching*, Pelham Books.

Maintenance Exercise Programme

General stretches for the lower back, hips and legs

This group of stretches will also help the muscles and joints of the hips, groin and hamstrings.

Many people still use the traditional technique of touching the toes to achieve a stretch and warm up for the lower back, hips and legs. If you are not suffering from any form of back problem, then this may be satisfactory, but should still be performed with caution.

My own view is that bending to touch the toes is inherently bad for anyone with back injuries. It strains the ligaments of the lower back, compresses the inter-vertebral discs unevenly and sometimes encourages disc material to compress the spinal nerves; yet it is really only much good at stretching your hamstrings and there are better ways to achieve longer hamstrings, as described in **Exercise 2** and **Exercise 6**.

1 CALF STRETCH

 To stretch the back of the lower leg.

- Stand facing a wall at a comfortable distance.

- Rest your forearms on the wall and your head on your arms.

- Place your right leg behind you, keeping it straight, foot flat.

- Move your left foot towards the wall and bend your left knee.

- With a straight back, move your hips to the wall.

- Hold for 20 seconds, relax and repeat three times.

- Repeat the exercise with the opposite leg.

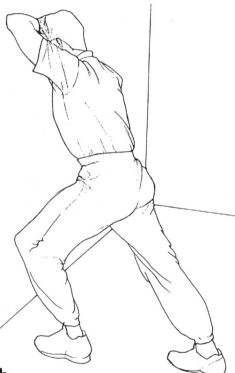

 If you do not feel the stretch, move your right foot slightly further from the wall.

2 HAMSTRING STRETCH

 To stretch the back of the upper leg.

- Sit with your legs straight, together or slightly apart.

- Keep your back straight.

- Bend forwards from the hip until you feel a tightness behind the knees.

- Hold for 20 seconds, relax and repeat three times.

- As you improve, try grasping your ankles. This allows you to relax and get a better stretch.

 You may find it easier to try this exercise sitting against a wall so that your back is held flat.

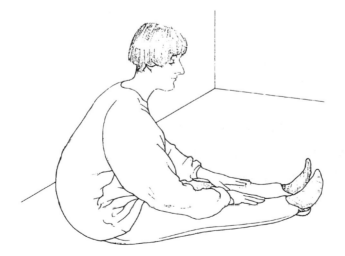

Alternative (1)

- Stand with one leg straight and the other leg raised up on a low platform, such as a foot-stool.

- Stand close to a wall or some stable object so that you can hold on.

- Keep your back straight.

- Bend from the hip until you feel a tightness behind the knee.

- Hold for 20 seconds, relax and repeat three times.

 Avoid any pulling sensation in the lower back — this suggests that you are letting the back bend or that too much effort is being used.

Alternative (2)*

- Sit with your legs straight, together or slightly apart.

- Keep your back straight.

- Loop a towel or scarf around your feet, keeping hold of the ends. This allows you to relax but does not strain the lower back.

- Bend forwards from the hip until you feel a tightness behind the knee.

- Hold for 20 seconds, relax and repeat three times.

- As you improve, try grasping your ankles. This allows you to relax and get a better stretch.

 You may find it easier to try this exercise sitting against a wall so that your back is held flat.

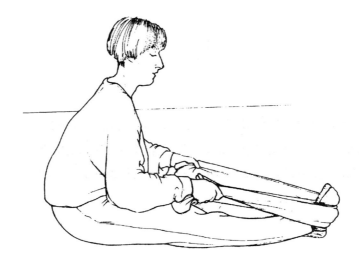

*This exercise is adapted from Bob Anderson (1981): *Stretching*, Pelham Books.

3 GROIN STRETCH

 To stretch the groin and inner thighs.

- Sit with the soles of your feet together, both knees fully bent.

- Lean gently forward and grasp your feet, but avoid bending your back.

- Pull yourself forward, using your feet as the anchor, until you feel a stretch in your groin and inner thighs.

- Hold for 20 seconds, relax and repeat three times.

 Increase the length of hold if you feel comfortable.

 To increase the stretch as you improve, use one hand to gently press down on one thigh.

 You may find it easier to try this exercise sitting against a wall so that your back is held flat.

4 LOWER-BACK STRETCH

 The groin-stretch position, as described in Exercise 3, is initially difficult for some people, but it does help to improve mobility in the lower back as well as stretch the groin muscles. In the position described next, it is not necessary to keep the soles of your feet together.

- Sit in a comfortable, cross-legged position.

- Lean forward from your hips and gently stretch your upper body towards the floor.

- Use your forearms in front of you to provide extra support.

- Hold this position for 20 seconds, sit up again and repeat three times.

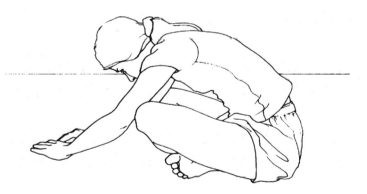

5 HIP AND THIGH STRETCH (LATERAL)

 To stretch the outer thigh and mobilise the hips. This stretch also helps the back of the arms and the waist.

- Sit with your left leg straight.

- Stabilise yourself with your right arm slightly behind you.

- Cross your right leg over the left so that the right foot is level with your left knee.

- Twist gently so that your left elbow rests outside the right knee.

- Using your left elbow, push your right knee across your body, from right to left.

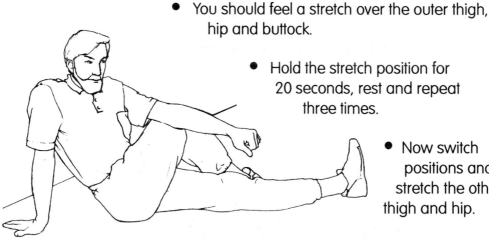

- You should feel a stretch over the outer thigh, hip and buttock.

- Hold the stretch position for 20 seconds, rest and repeat three times.

- Now switch positions and stretch the other thigh and hip.

 Twisting your trunk will increase the stretch, but be careful to avoid excessive stretching of the lower back.

6 KNEE TO CHEST

 To isolate one leg at a time for specific hamstring, buttock and lower-back stretching.

- Roll onto your back.

- Slowly bend one knee and slide your foot towards your bottom, so that your knee is bent.

- Reach forward with both hands, clasp your knee and link your fingers together.

- Gently pull the knee towards your chest and then relax for a moment.

- Once relaxed, pull the knee in further until the back of your thigh and your lower back feel a stretch.

- Hold for 20 seconds, rest and repeat three times.

- Repeat for the other leg.

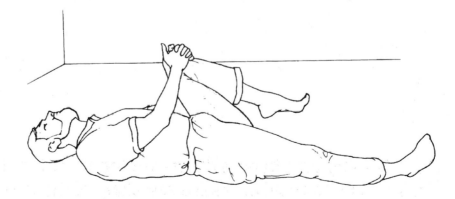

7 PELVIC TILTING

 This is a nice relaxing stretch that even the stiffest people can attempt and one which greatly helps the junction of the spine and pelvis.

- Lie on your back and draw both knees up.

- Let your arms rest away from your body for stability.

- Keep the same position and tilt your pelvis backwards so that the small of the back presses gently onto the floor.

- Hold each tilt for five seconds, relax and repeat up to 20 times.

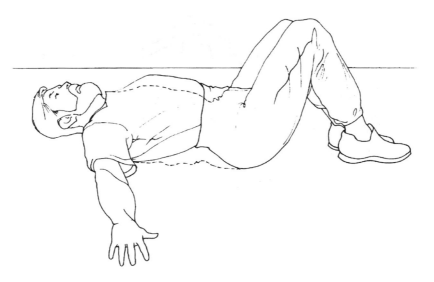

 The number of repetitions can be increased at will as long as no pain is felt.

8 ROLL-UP

 This exercise helps as a general stretcher of the whole back and can be very comforting.

- Make sure that you are on a soft surface like a rug.

- Sit up and hug both knees.

- Gently roll onto your back and rock back and forth.

- If you find this comfortable, repeat at will.

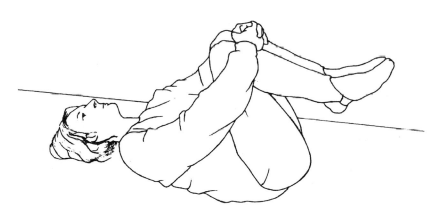

9 SQUATTING

- Simple squatting can be of great help in stretching your lower back and calves, whatever your state of health. You will feel stretch in the back, buttocks, ankles and Achilles tendons.

- Squat down keeping the feet flat, both for stability and ankle stretching.

- Hold for 20 seconds or as long as you are comfortable.

- If you find it easier, squat so that your back is up against a wall, lending you support.

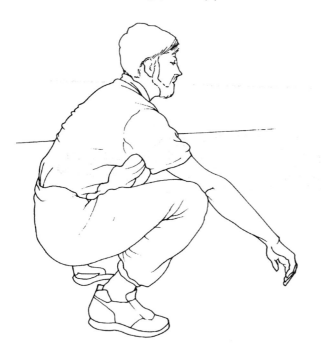

 Avoid this exercise if you have injuries to the cartilages in your knees or have replacement joints in your knees or hips.

10 LONG STRETCH

 To stretch the long tissues that run throughout the body.

- Lie on your back.

- Extend your arms and legs.

- Reach as far as you can with your fingers and toes in opposite directions.

- Hold for five seconds, relax and repeat three times.

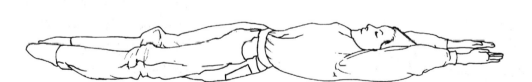

11 SIDE-BEND STRETCH

 To stretch the long tissues of the flanks and the back of the arm.

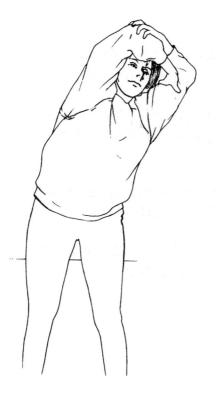

- Stand with legs comfortably apart, knees slightly bent.

- Fold your arms above your head, loosely holding the opposite elbow of each arm.

- Bend gently left and pull on the right elbow at the same time.

- Hold for 15 seconds. Relax and straighten, repeat three times.

- Repeat, bending to the right.

12 OVERHEAD STRETCH

 To stretch the tissues of the back and under the arms.

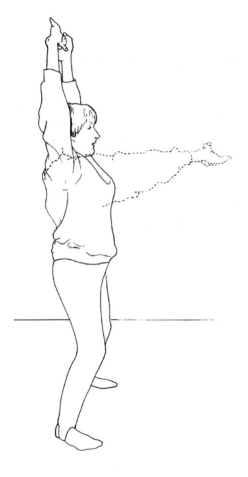

- Stand with legs comfortably apart, knees slightly bent.

- Lace fingers together, and push your palms outward in front of you.

- Stretch straight arms above your head and reach upwards.

- Hold for 15 seconds. Relax and repeat three times.

13 HIP AND THIGH STRETCH (FRONT)

 To stretch the hip and the muscles at the front of the thigh.

- Kneel on your right knee, so that it is slightly behind you.

- Bend your left leg so that your foot is flat and your left knee is over the left ankle.

- Allow your left knee to bend and your hips to lower to the floor so that a stretch develops in the right thigh.

- Hold for 20 seconds, relax and repeat three times with each leg.

This exercise is particularly helpful for those with lower-back pain or postural problems. This is because a powerful muscle that extends from the front of the lumbar spine, through the abdomen and into the thigh is stretched, relieving muscular constraints on the spine.

14 QUADRICEPS STRETCH

 This exercise complements the hamstring stretch described in Exercise 2 by stretching the front of the thigh.

- Stand facing a wall, placing your left hand on it for support.

- Reach down and behind you with your right hand and grasp your left leg at the ankle.

- Gently pull your heel towards your buttock.

- Hold for 20 seconds, relax and repeat three times

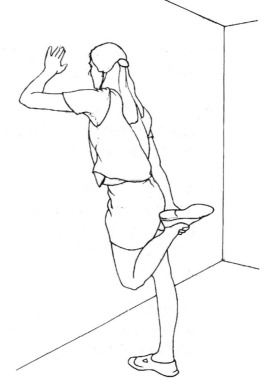

15 TOWEL STRETCH

 To stretch the tissues of the breast and shoulders.

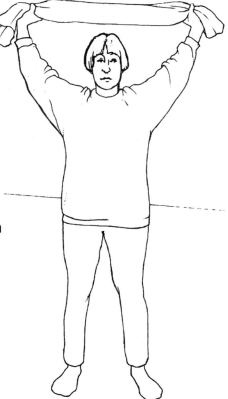

- Stand with legs comfortably apart, knees slightly bent.

- Hold a large towel at both ends.

- Straighten both arms in front of you and move them apart so that the towel is taut.

- Lift your arms above your head and as far behind you as you can manage comfortably.

- Hold for 15 seconds, relax and repeat five times.

 If your hands are far enough apart, you will be able to roll your shoulders so that your arms pass behind you.

16 STOMACH CURL (QUARTER SIT-UP)

 To warm up the lower stomach and thigh muscles.

 This is not a full sit-up. Just head and shoulders off the floor.

- Lie on your back with your knees bent and feet flat on the floor or against a wall as shown in the illustration.

- Place your hands beside you, palms downwards and breathe in deeply.

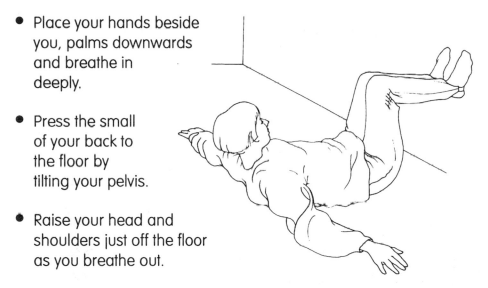

- Press the small of your back to the floor by tilting your pelvis.

- Raise your head and shoulders just off the floor as you breathe out.

- Hold this position for a second and then relax back as you breathe in again.

- Carry out ten repetitions.

 To begin with, increase repetitions slowly by one or two repetitions per day.

Exercise Guide for Maintenance Plan

To use this guide (and those in the sections that follow) choose the area of your body that you wish to influence and refer to the numbered exercise. How long you choose to keep doing these or any other exercises will depend how much time you have available and how fit you wish to be.

None of the exercises requires special equipment and all can be performed selectively although the intention is that they follow a sensible sequence. Perhaps you might want to concentrate on the lower body on Monday, Wednesday and Friday and the upper body on Tuesday, Thursday and Saturday; the lower back and abdomen can be covered six days a week and take Sunday off as a reward!

Please remember that these exercises are not designed to become a burden to you; they should help you personally and the one for whom you care. There is no obligation and, if you only have time to select a few that seem most relevant and do them on alternate days, then doing some exercise some of the time is better than doing none at all.

Target Area	Stretch name and number	Page number	How long & how many	Frequency
Lower leg	Calf Stretch (1)	38	20 secs. x 3	3 x per week
Upper leg	Hamstring (2)	39	20 secs. x 3	3 x per week
Hips and Thighs	Hip & Thigh Stretch (lateral) (5)	44	20 secs. x 3	3 x per week
	Hip & Thigh Stretch (front) (13)	52	20 secs. x 3	3 x per week
	Quadriceps Stretch (14)	53	20 secs. x 3	3 x per week
Groin	Groin Stretch (3)	42	20 secs. x 3	3 x per week
Stomach (Abdomen)	Stomach Curl (16)	55	10 x	6 x per week
Lower Back	Lower-back Stretch (4)	43	15 secs. x 3	6 x per week
	Knee-to-chest (6)	45	20 secs. x 3	6 x per week
	Pelvic Tilting (7)	46	5 secs. x 3	6 x per week
	Squatting (9)	48	20–60 secs	6 x per week
Whole Back	Roll-up (8)	47	At will	6 x per week
Whole Body	Long Stretch (10)	49	5 secs. x 3	3 x per week
Flanks and Arms	Side-bend Stretch (11)	50	15 secs. x 3	3 x per week
	Overhead Stretch (12)	51	15 secs. x 3	3 x per week
Shoulders and Chest	Towel Stretch (15)	54	15 secs. x 5	3 x per week

Keeping Healthy

Sport differs from exercise. Use the exercises and stretches in the **Maintenance Exercise Programme** to gain some basic fitness before you start doing an organised sport. This applies both to those who are recovering from an injury and to those simply unused to exercise. Taking up a sport can, however, improve the speed at which you recover when sport and exercise are sensibly combined.

- Make sure that you are wearing appropriate clothing for the sport that you choose.

- If you buy treadmills, rowing or cycling machines, make sure that they are what you need. Don't just take up a sport because you think it is 'good for you'.

- Do something you enjoy so that expensive equipment does not end up in the loft.

- Many Sports Centres now have their own physiotherapist or osteopath. Ask them for advice on the best sports for you.

Upper body

Hand or wrist **weights** are good for toning arms and shoulders, while also helping the neck. Buy light weights to start with and build up slowly. Twenty repetitions with a half or 1kg. (1–2lb.) weight is generally better than five repetitions with a 4.5kg. (10lb.) weight.

'Resistance' bands are available. These are long, colourful elastic bands several centimetres wide and of varying levels of resistance. They are particularly useful for building strength and stamina after shoulder injuries.

Whole body

Push-pull type **exercise-bikes** tone the whole body, while **rowing machines** may aggravate lower-back strains.

Swimming is generally accepted as one of the best all-round exercises. Avoid breast-stroke if you have suffered an upper-back or neck injury but substitute with backstroke or sidestroke.

Walking is a good aerobic exercise if done briskly. Keep on level ground.

Aerobics

If you want to take up aerobics as a way to help you recover from an injury, wait until any pain is gone. Aerobic exercise classes are very popular but are physically demanding. Much of the routine is done standing, jogging and jumping and is stressful to the lower back and leg joints. Find a qualified instructor in **low-impact** aerobics. If you have had any injuries, make sure your instructor knows about them. Wait out those movements that cause any discomfort.

Step-aerobics calls for strong leg, back and abdominal muscles, as well as stamina. Keep your exercise routine simple at first and start to use the more technical steps as your fitness improves. Keep the step at the right height for you.

Be cautious of the degree of twisting and pelvic tilting that is an inevitable part of this very popular form of exercise, as it can be hard on the lower back in particular.

Jogging

If you want to start jogging as a way to help you recover after an injury, wait until any pain is gone. This is especially important if you have had leg or lower-back injuries. Even if you have very good technique, this sport is stressful on the lower body. If you are a slogger rather than a jogger, you can do more harm to your body than good. Run on dry grass rather than metalled roads or pavements where possible. After you finish your jog, warm down for several minutes before stopping.

Swimming

Swimming is probably the most popular and accessible form of exercise for many people. It is something that can be done alone, but one has the feeling of being in company, unlike jogging. You can do it gently or vigorously and one does not have to have an excellent technique.

Be cautious of breast-stroke if you have a neck or upper-back strain. Unless you can swim with your head down in the water, lifting your head back can cause further strain.

Exercise guide for selected sports

Choose the area or activity you wish to improve. Specific sports covered by the exercises and stretches in this book are shown by name, exercise number and page number. Remember this is only a guide and it is preferable that you do as many of the stretches as you can manage. Do not continue with any form of exercise or stretch if you experience pain.

Target Area	Stretch name and number	Page number	How long & how many
Aerobics	Calf Stretch (1)	38	20 secs. x 3
	Hamstring Stretch (2)	39	20 secs. x 3
	Groin Stretch (3)	42	20 secs. x 3
	Lower-back Stretch (4)	43	20 secs. x 3
	Hip and Thigh Stretch (Lateral) (5)	44	20 secs. x 3
	Knee-to-chest (6)	45	20 secs. x 3
	Pelvic Tilting (7)	46	5 secs. x 20
	Side-bend Stretch (11)	50	15 secs. x 3
	Overhead Stretch (12)	51	15 secs. x 3
	Hip and Thigh Stretch (Front) (13)	52	20 secs. x 3
	Quadriceps Stretch (14)	53	20 secs. x 3
	Stomach Curl (16)	55	10 x
Jogging	Calf Stretch (1)	38	20 secs. x 3
	Hamstring Stretch (2)	39	20 secs. x 3
	Groin Stretch (3)	42	20 secs. x 3
	Hip and Thigh Stretch (Lateral) (5)	44	20 secs. x 3
	Squatting (9)	48	20 secs. x 3
Swimming	Groin Stretch (3)	42	20 secs. x 3
	Hip and Thigh Stretch (Lateral) (5)	44	20 secs. x 3
	Squatting (9)	48	20 secs. x 3
	Long Stretch (10)	49	5 secs. x 20
	Side-bend Stretch (11)	50	15 secs. x 3
	Overhead Stretch (12)	51	15 secs. x 3
	Hip and Thigh Stretch (Front) (13)	52	20 secs. x 3
	Towel Stretch (15)	54	15 secs. x 3
	Stomach Curl (16)	55	10 x

Relaxation

Most of us would agree with the truism that we live in a society where stress is endemic and yet we tend to react poorly when it is suggested that stress affects *us*. We tend to see only the negative aspects of stress, yet we need to accept that not only is stress around us constantly, but stress is also necessary, both physiologically and emotionally.

The term 'psychosomatic' is defined as: 'referring to the relationship between mind and body'*. This tells us that the mind has a direct influence upon the body. It does not suggest that a stress-related illness is 'all in the mind', the interpretation that is sadly so often put upon it nowadays, nor that a physical pain is being imagined.

Both emotional and physical stresses can affect our health directly. Exercise as a physical stress is usually seen as positive, but overdo it and we become injured. The same can be said if we give too much emotionally to our charges. A carer who is tired and emotionally taxed is, in my view, more likely to suffer injury; it is, therefore, important that we know how to relax.

I state again that a carer has a duty to care both for themselves and for the person in their care. If a little selfishness in the short term helps us to cope better in the future, that benefits everyone. Although the term is incompatible with itself, I am advocating a little selfish altruism; take the **Duty of Care** principle and treat it holistically.

*Churchill's Medical Dictionary.

Use relaxation tapes, yoga, meditation, religion; the responsibility is your own to find what suits you best. I admire those who can lie on a floor and imagine the tension out of their muscles and float their troubles away, but it is not for everyone.

Many patients relax so well that they almost go to sleep on the treatment couch. The therapist often rightly gets the credit, but I believe that for many people the chance to lie down in peace and quiet during a busy day, with someone looking after *them*, is a huge part of the effect. Note the rise in interest in aromatherapy over the last few years.

For those who find it difficult to relax physically, indulge yourself in an absorbing hobby or activity so that your mind is refreshed.

If an Injury Occurs

Self-Help and First Aid

Whether you need expert help after an injury or feel you can manage yourself, first aid and self-help techniques can help you improve more quickly.

Assess the extent of the injury. If you fall over, don't leap to your feet, embarrassed and flustered; literally search your body for damage before getting up.

Lower back

- Regain composure and take a deep breath. Look for pain in the back, tingling or numbness in the legs.

- If you find any of these, call for help as you *may* have a spinal disc injury.

- **Ice-packs help to reduce swelling**. A large packet of frozen peas wrapped in a tea-towel and placed over the painful area is the easiest method. Leave this on for about ten minutes but avoid direct contact of the packet with your skin.

- In the early stages after an injury, the application of heat, whilst comforting, encourages swelling; this ultimately creates stiffness and more pain.

- When lying on your side, draw your knees up slightly and place a pillow between them to reduce any twist on the spine.

- Avoid massage in acute muscle spasm as this can aggravate.

- Often in lower-back pain, most comfort is found on the floor, lying on your side. Beds can be too soft and do not give good support. If lying flat is more comfortable, then do it!

- Try to keep a phone within reach while recovering.

- Avoid propping your head up for too long — don't add neck strain to your situation.

- Forget the vacuuming, gardening and ironing — you may *have* to collect the children from school but most other 'obligations' can wait.

- Once the initial pain has settled, occasional movement is desirable. Go to the toilet, make a cup of tea or simply turn over. Try to do something every hour.

- Start using the exercise regime only when pain has subsided. If unsure when to start, ask your GP or other health professional.

Neck and shoulders

First aid for shoulder strains usually involves rest and using some form of ice-pack. Ice-packs are simple, safe and help to reduce swelling, bruising and pain.

Massage, heat, cold, traction and manipulation all have their place in neck injuries but have to be used selectively and you must get good, professional advice. If you are prescribed a rigid support collar, avoid driving or operating machinery.

If the onset of pain is rapid, neck and shoulder injuries are fairly easy to judge. However, many neck and shoulder pains start more gradually and some of these fall into the category of overuse injuries, which are often called Repetitive Strain Injuries (RSI), or Upper Limb Disorder (ULD). If your injury is in this category, you will need to examine how you lift and work to see how you can alleviate the causes of your problem, as well as take steps to have your problem treated.

- Check for dizziness and tingling, numbness or weakness in the arms, as well as pain. If you experience any of these symptoms, call your doctor.

- Ice-packs are preferable to heat, as with most acute injuries.

- Support your neck by wrapping a towel or rolled newspaper around it. **Do not wrap anything too tightly around your neck**; leave sufficient room to allow you to breathe freely, and for some limited movement.

- Avoid driving, washing your hair, lifting — anything that means you have to bend or turn your head.

- Shoulders need to be rested initially and a sling reminds you not to use the injured arm. Put on a jacket and ask someone to pin the open front to the lapel, wrapping the arm and elbow as you do so.

Start exercises only after the pain has settled or on specialist advice.

Course of a typical injury to the lumbar spine

Perhaps the most frequently asked question that I hear is, 'How long is this going to take to get better?' The main concern for most patients, whether self-employed or employed, is that of getting back to work as soon as possible. It doesn't matter whether that work is a conventional paid job or whether they have responsibilities in the home, this question almost always comes to the fore.

The most common injuries that I as an osteopath am consulted about are those to the lower part of the back. The commonest history that these patients give is much as follows:

'All I did was reach down to put on my socks and I felt something give in my back. It didn't particularly hurt, but I knew something was wrong. By the end of the day, my back was very stiff and painful and I could only get comfortable lying on the floor.'

The injury is often so simple, that the sufferer may not even associate the event with the pain that follows. The position that is most often responsible for the injury is a combination movement that involves bending (forwards or backwards) and twisting to one side. Other examples are: vacuum-cleaning, helping someone out of a chair, a driver reaching for a briefcase from the back seat of the car, and lifting a small child out of a cot that is in an awkward corner.

The graph opposite shows the typical length of time that a moderate-to-severe lumbar injury takes to resolve. This is the type of injury that is most commonly experienced, where muscles and joints are sprained, forcing them beyond their normal limits. Such injuries *do not* include lumbar disc **prolapse**, which is a much more serious event. You will find more information on the 'slipped disc' in the next section on page 70.

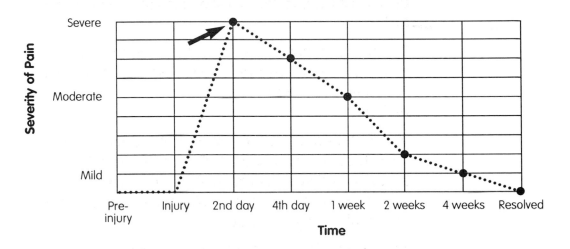

Graphical Representation of Pain versus Time for Lumbar Disc/Joint Injury

The arrow depicts the point at which many people decide to call for assistance. By the second day after the injury, pain has often *increased* and this frequently triggers a call from the patient to their GP or osteopath asking for treatment. Pain will gradually diminish over the next two days, accelerating in improvement towards the end of the first week. By the end of the second week, the injury should have reached the stage where it does not interfere too much with normal activity. By week four, you will probably find that you only think about your injury if someone asks, or after a heavy day.

People, of course, vary a great deal; some will improve faster, others will find it takes six to eight weeks before they feel that the problem has resolved. The extent of the injury and the speed with which you get treatment are the determining factors. Inevitably, if the injury is several weeks old by the time you take remedial action, then the recovery period is extended.

When to treat?

The best time to treat is on the second or third day after injury, when the swelling that takes place around the site of the injury has reached its maximum and then begun to subside. This often seems rather unkind to the sufferer who, quite reasonably, wants to be seen as soon as humanly possible.

However, as with any medical condition, there are exceptions. Make an appointment to see your GP, osteopath or physiotherapist, if you need advice on how severe your injury is. The point is that they may well be able to begin treatment with advice, electrotherapy or medication where appropriate. Actual manual treatment such as massage, manipulation, traction or exercise may not be beneficial at this stage, if at all, but at least the process has been started.

Those fortunate people who never experience back pain cannot understand, however sympathetic they may be, the level of discomfort and the depressing quality that it can bring.

The 'slipped' disc

The slipped disc is more properly known as a **prolapsed** or **herniated** disc. The term 'slipped' seems to imply that the disc has moved out of its normal position, rather like a coin pokes out of a stack of change, and that it can simply be slipped back in again. This quite inaccurate impression is very widespread and understates the severe nature of this type of injury.

In reality, a prolapsed or 'slipped' disc is an escape of the soft *nucleus pulposus* from its 'container', the fibrous outer part of the disc, pushing both fibrous and nucleus material onto sensitive tissues like the nerves. The inner disc material uses a weak area in the wall of the fibrous part to escape.

Disc prolapses can occur anywhere in the spinal column, but the most common site of a prolapse is in the lumbar spine. The prolapse most often takes place at the back of the disc, usually to one side or the other, but occasionally directly backwards. A prolapse may happen as a result of accidents to the spine, or repeated postural or occupational stresses, or inherited weakness of the disc material. Of course, any combination of these will increase the risk of prolapse.

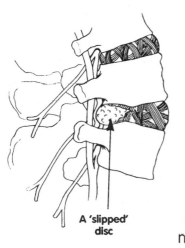

A 'slipped' disc

The direction in which the prolapse takes place is an important point to consider, because this will affect the symptoms that are experienced. If the prolapse is onto the *right* nerve root, then the sufferer will experience sciatic pain in the right leg. If the prolapse is to the *left*, the left sciatic nerve is affected. Should the pressure be directly backwards onto the spinal cord, then sciatica is felt in *both* legs.

Sciatica is a symptom of lumbar disc injury. Pain is felt in the back of the thigh and may continue into the calf, ankle or even foot. It becomes very difficult to lift your leg when lying down and is a most demoralising type of pain. One test that is used is Straight Leg Raising, where the patient lies on their back and lifts one leg as far as possible, without bending their knee. The test is repeated for both legs. Sharp pain down the line of the sciatic nerve after only a few degrees of lift is indicative of prolapsed inter-vertebral disc.

Happily, however, 'true' sciatica from a prolapsed disc is relatively uncommon, even though it is often suggested as an initial diagnosis.

Bulging, where disc material deforms the disc and yet does not prolapse, is, in my opinion, far more common. Symptoms may well be similar to those of prolapse but settle much more readily, responding well to exercises designed to reduce muscle spasm and pressure around the injury.

Sciatic symptoms can also be caused by muscle spasm in the lower back and buttock; this is often dismissed as 'only muscular'.

Here is a basic checklist of symptoms. You must seek a professional opinion if you are experiencing any of these:

● pain in the back of the thigh, calf, ankle and under the foot which could be described as sharp, tingling, burning, aching or stabbing;

● pain that is constant, whatever your position;

● an inability to raise your leg off the bed;

● frequency of passing water.

I would suggest the following while you wait for attention:

● Do *not* apply heat to your lower back.

● You can apply an **ice-pack** to your lower back. Leave it on for ten minutes only, but you can re-apply every hour. Remember to prevent the ice-pack touching your skin directly, by wrapping it in, for example, a tea-towel.

● Find a comfortable position; this may be lying flat on your back, or on your side with a pillow between your knees.

● Change position every thirty to forty minutes, so that you do not 'set'.

● Get your GP's advice *before* you take painkillers, as he or she might choose to give you a different prescription.

Self-Help Exercise Programmes

Prevention or maintenance?

The relevance of the recovery programmes which follow remains the same whether you are looking to strengthen your body to *prevent* injury or to *recover* from injury — the factor that changes is the speed with which you can increase the frequency of exercise and the number of repetitions of each one.

Precautions

- If you do have an injury, exercises should only be begun once any acute pain has settled. Typically, this will be three to five days after you have hurt yourself. After an injury, exercise may cause a slight initial increase in pain. This is quite normal and will usually not be noticed after the first few sets of exercise.

- If an injury is serious, most people are able to decide that this is the case and will call medical attention immediately. When the problem is less clear cut, the decision to call for help is more difficult. **If in doubt, call!**

- You may wish to seek professional advice from your GP, osteopath, chartered or state-registered physiotherapist or chiropractor before beginning these recovery programmes.

- *You* ultimately have responsibility for your own health. If you decide to manage the injury yourself, it is still wise to seek qualified advice.

The exercises in the self-help programmes should be performed once or twice a day, depending upon your fitness and flexibility. Whether you have an injury or not, begin by doing the exercises as described below once or twice a day for one week before trying to increase the number of repetitions or the number of sessions.

It is far safer to take things slowly. Make the exercises part of your daily routine and then you won't be put off by trying too hard, perhaps slowing your recovery and then stopping altogether.

Recovery Programme for Back Pain and Injuries

Most of these techniques are what I would describe as active exercises, which means that your muscles and joints are put through a range of movements that may be beyond what you normally experience. For the otherwise healthy individual, this does not present any difficulty and will cause only the sort of mild aches that always accompany new activity.

Week One: Stretch and strengthen

Lying on your front

17 PRE-EXERCISE RELAXATION

 For relaxation and preparation prior to your exercises.

- Lie face down or on one side, making sure that your head is comfortable.

- The position is not very important since the aim is to be able to relax.

- Breathe evenly and relax for two minutes, allowing any muscle spasm to settle.

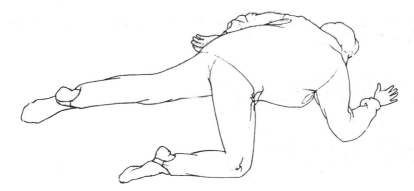

 If you lie on your front, you may find it more comfortable with a small pillow under your lower abdomen or hips.

18 PRONE EXTENSION A

 To gently mobilise and stretch, especially the lumbar spine.

 This is not a press up.

If you have been lying on your side, roll onto your front, remove the pillow if this was used, and relax again for a few seconds.

- Place your hands, palms down, under your shoulders and breathe slowly in.

- As you breathe out, using only arm and shoulder power, push up until you feel your hips begin to ease off the floor.

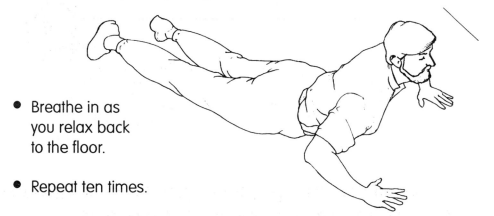

- Breathe in as you relax back to the floor.

- Repeat ten times.

- Relax for a minute before the next exercise.

 At each repetition you should stretch back a little further, but never let your hips off the floor.

19 PRONE EXTENSION B

 To help regain muscle tone and strength.

- Stay on your front and put your hands down by your sides, palms upwards.

- Breathe out and gently raise your head and shoulders off the floor.

- Hold this position for a second and then relax back to the floor, breathing in as you go.

- Perform ten repetitions and then rest for a minute.

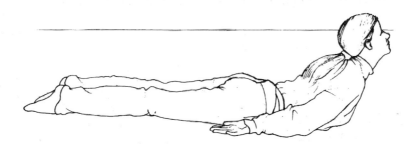

 As you get stronger, move your hand position from by your sides into the small of your back.

 Moving your hand position can put more strain on the lower-back muscles and should not be attempted until the second week of the Recovery Programme, if discomfort is felt.

Lying on your back

20 KNEE-TO-CHEST A

 To stretch the lower spine and strengthen the stomach muscles.

- Strong stomach muscles help to take some strain off your back. Your stomach muscles play an important part in supporting your trunk in general. These muscles often become fatigued, especially if you have suffered from a lower-back injury. If the stomach muscles are healthy and strong, they will help to maintain posture and take some strain off your back.

- Roll onto your back.

- Bend your left knee and slide your foot along the floor towards your bottom.

- Reach forward and clasp the knee.

- With fingers linked, gently pull the knee towards your chest and then relax for a moment.

- Pull your knee towards you gently twenty times, feeling a stretch in the lower back. Repeat with the right knee.

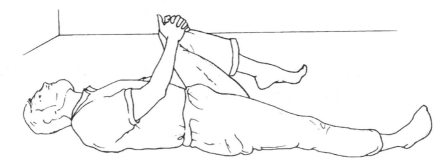

 Pull in your stomach muscles at the same time; this will also strengthen the waist.

21 LUMBAR ROTATION A

 To increase mobility in the hips and lower back.

- Stay on your back with knees comfortably bent and your feet flat against the floor.

- Let your arms rest away from your body, with your palms downwards, for stability.

- Keep your knees together, and let your knees fall to each side in turn, 15–20 times.

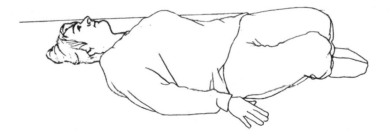

 Allow a rhythm to develop and momentum will do much of the work.

22 STOMACH CURL (QUARTER-SIT-UP)

This is a repeat of **Exercise 16** but fits in well at this point in the **Recovery Programme**.

 To further strengthen the lower stomach and thigh muscles.

 This is not a full sit-up. Only head and shoulders off the floor.

- Stay on your back with knees bent and feet flat against the floor.

- Place your hands beside you, palms downwards, and breathe deeply.

- Press the small of your back towards the floor by tilting your pelvis.

- Raise your head and shoulders just off the floor as you breathe out.

- Hold this position for a second and then relax back as you breathe in again.

- Carry out ten repetitions.

- Stay at ten repetitions of this exercise once a day for one week before increasing the number of repetitions, or moving on to **Exercise 29** in **Week Two**.

 When you do increase the number of repetitions, do so by one or two repetitions per day.

On all fours

23 KNEELING ARCH A

 To increase the mobility of the whole spine.

 It is most important that the whole spine is arched to protect the base of the neck. Avoid bending the neck beyond what feels comfortable. This is particularly important for the elderly and those with circulatory problems or rheumatoid arthritis.

- From lying on your back, gently roll first onto your side, and then come up onto all fours.

- Allow your back to sag, and relax in this position for a few seconds.

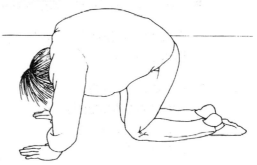

- With one smooth movement, pull your head and neck gently downwards towards the floor and arch your spine.

- Slowly reverse your position, allowing your back to sag and bending your head slightly backwards .

- Repeat this exercise 15 to 20 times.

The seven exercises that comprise **Week One** of the **Recovery Programme** should be performed twice a day (apart from **Exercise 22**, where once a day is sufficient). When you can perform them comfortably, you are ready to move on to **Week Two** of the **Recovery Programme**. It is not, however, obligatory that exactly seven days after starting the programme, you move on. You are an individual, with a specific set of needs, and if it takes ten days to feel comfortable, then this is perfectly all right.

Week Two: Increasing your strength

The point at which you are ready to start this sequence of exercises will depend on your initial fitness and the severity of your injury. Therefore, please remember that some individuals may need to carry on with '**Week One**' for a further few days; others will feel able to start these exercises sooner. If you have any doubts, please seek professional advice. Some of the exercises are extensions of those you now know, others are new.

Lying on your front

24 PRE-EXERCISE RELAXATION

 For relaxation and preparation prior to your exercises. Start all your exercise sessions by relaxing and preparing your mind and body.

- Lie face down or on one side, making sure that your head is comfortable.

- The position is not very important since the aim is to be able to relax.

- Breathe evenly and relax for two minutes. This gives time for muscle spasm to settle.

 If you lie on your front, you may find it more comfortable with a small pillow under your lower abdomen or hips.

25 PRONE EXTENSION A

 To gently stretch and mobilise the whole spine, especially the lumbar section.

 This is a repeat of Exercise 18 but remember, it is still not a press up.

- If you have been lying on your side, roll onto your front, remove the pillow if this was used, and relax again for a few seconds.

- Place your hands under your shoulders and breathe slowly in.

- As you breathe out, using only arm and shoulder power, push up until you feel your hips begin to ease off the floor.

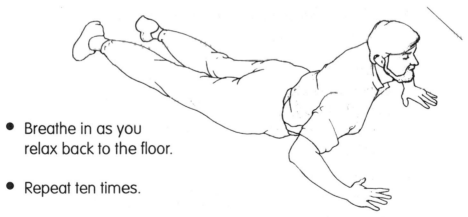

- Breathe in as you relax back to the floor.

- Repeat ten times.

- Relax for a minute before the next exercise.

 At each repetition you should stretch back a little further, but never let your hips off the floor.

26 PRONE EXTENSION C

For progressive strengthening of your back muscles.

- Stay on your front but this time cup your hands into the small of your back.

- Squeeze your knees and feet together.

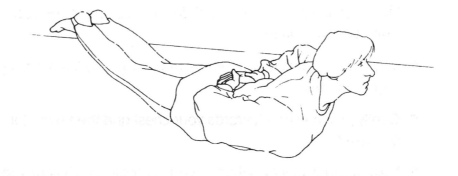

- Breathe in and then, as you exhale, lift both legs together just off the floor, while raising your head and shoulders.

- Hold this position for a second, then slowly lower your legs, head and shoulders until your body is flat.

- Repeat ten times.

Lying on your back

27 KNEE-TO-CHEST B

 To stretch the lower spine and, indirectly, to strengthen the stomach muscles. Please note that this exercise is in two parts and extends the difficulty of Exercise 20.

Part 1

- Roll from your front onto your back.

- Slowly bend your knees and slide your feet along the floor towards your bottom.

- Reach forward with both hands and clasp one knee, linking fingers in front.

- Gently pull the knee towards your chest and then relax for a moment.

- Next, using about one third of your strength, push your knee away from you but hold it firmly so that it does not move.

- Keep the pressure on for five seconds and then relax.

- Now pull your knee closer to your chest and repeat the push.

- Do this three times with each knee, and then three times with both knees together.

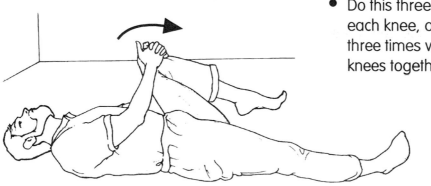

Part 2

- Put your feet back onto the floor and let your arms rest away from your body for stability.

- Keeping in this same position, tilt your pelvis backwards so that the small of your back presses gently onto the floor.

- Perform twenty repetitions. You can increase this number at will as long as no pain is felt.

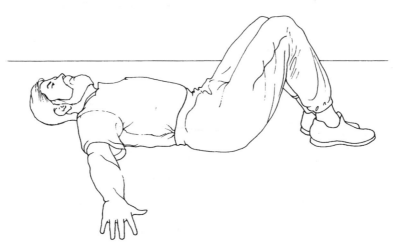

 Pull in your stomach muscles at the same time as you tilt your pelvis. This assists the exercise and also strengthens the waist.

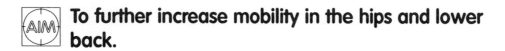

28 LUMBAR ROTATION B

 To further increase mobility in the hips and lower back.

- Lie on your back with your knees comfortably bent, feet flat against the floor, and legs held together.

- Let your knees fall to each side in turn 15–20 times.

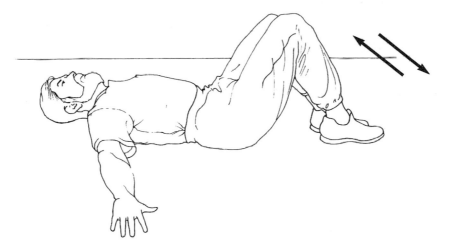

Perform the side-to-side movement more slowly than in Week One so that the effort is greater.

29 STOMACH CURL (ADVANCED QUARTER-SIT-UP)

 To further strengthen the lower-stomach and thigh muscles.

The difficulty is increased slightly by placing your hands at head level rather than on the floor beside you; this makes the top half of your body heavier. Also, you may now feel that you are ready to place your feet up against a wall, as shown in the illustration.

 This is not a full sit-up. If your lower back feels strained, you may be lifting your head and shoulders too high off the floor.

- Stay on your back with knees bent and feet flat against the floor.

- Place your hands over your ears.

- Press the small of your back towards the floor by tilting your pelvis. Raise your head and shoulders off the floor, as you breathe out.

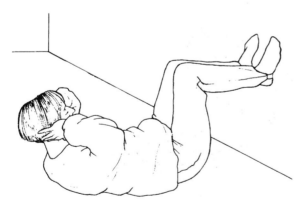

- Hold this position for a second and then relax back as you breathe in again.

- Carry out ten repetitions.

- Stay at ten repetitions of this exercise once a day for one further week before increasing the number of repetitions.

 When you do increase the number of repetitions, do so by one or two repetitions per day.

On all fours

30 KNEELING ARCH B

 To increase the mobility of the whole spine.

While initially similar to **Exercise 23**, this exercise increases your effort and strengthens the abdominal, thigh and buttock muscles as well as those of the lower back.

 Avoid bending the neck beyond what feels comfortable. This is particularly important for the elderly and those with circulatory problems or rheumatoid arthritis.

- From lying on your back, gently roll first onto your side, and then come onto all fours.

- Allow your back to sag, and relax in this position for a few seconds.

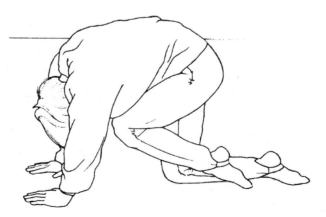

- In one movement, bend your head downwards, arch your back and bend one knee forward.

- Try to touch your forehead with your knee. (This is not essential, just a target to aim at.)

- Next, as you raise your head, stretch one leg out behind you.

- Combine these movements into a smooth sequence, then repeat the routine backwards and forwards ten times.

- Repeat with the other leg.

These seven exercises in **Week Two** of the **Recovery Programme** should be performed once or twice a day (apart from **Exercise 29**, which you should do once a day only). Do them for one week before trying to increase the number of repetitions or the number of sessions.

Recovery Programme for the Shoulders

Pains in the neck and shoulders come from a variety of sources. The shoulder in particular is something of a compromise joint. It has to be very mobile and powerful, while still staying stable. Perhaps more than any other joint in the body, the shoulders rely on the health and good functioning of the muscles and tendons that surround them. Some of the muscles in the neck that support the head and allow its movement, also play an important part in moving the shoulders.

Exercises that involve the neck and shoulders are important even if you have an injury to only one of those areas. The exercises that follow have names that relate to specific areas, but they will inevitably affect both neck and shoulders. I would recommend that you perform both sets of exercises.

Most of us do not use our shoulders throughout their full range, and so these exercises, though simple, are very useful in keeping the joints active. Do all of the exercises for the shoulders with *both* arms. This allows you to compare the two sides of your body and to monitor any improvement.

Even if you have no injuries, many of you will notice that one shoulder is more flexible than the other. The exercises that follow are therefore recommended as a valuable part of your daily routine; they are easily done almost anywhere and will help to keep your neck more supple as well as improve your shoulders.

31 SHOULDER ROTATION

 To reduce gently any stiffness and to prevent the muscles from weakening.

- Stand near a table or worktop that is stable.

- Bend gently forward at the waist and hold onto the table with the good arm.

- Allow your injured arm to dangle downward. You may wish to hold a small weight, but do not exceed 1kg (2.2lb).

- Swing your injured arm clockwise in small circles twenty times.

- Stop gently, reverse the direction and swing your arm anti-clockwise twenty times.

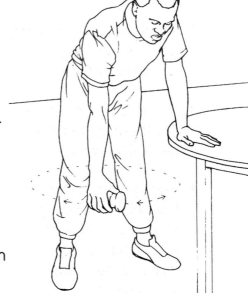

- Stop gently once again.

- Allow the arm to swing backwards and forwards, again twenty times. Stop gently.

- Finally, swing your arm across in front of your body for the same number of repetitions.

32 WALL-WALKING

 To increase the range of shoulder movement and prevent the joints from stiffening.

If you have normal shoulders, you should find no difficulty in doing this exercise, but it is very useful in providing a passive stretch to the muscles, tendons and joints. This exercise is therefore particularly useful for conditions like 'frozen shoulder', but will also help with a simple stiff shoulder joint.

- Place a chair at right angles about 30cm (21 inches) away from a wall.

- Sit down on the chair with the stiff or injured arm nearest the wall.

- Place your hand flat on the wall and, using your fingers, start to 'walk' your hand upwards as far as the shoulder will let you go.

- Let your arm slide back down.

- Repeat this ten times.

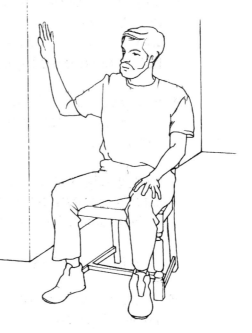

 Mark the wall at the highest point you reach. Beat it each day.

33 SHOULDER SWING

 To strengthen the shoulder muscles.

- Stand comfortably with your back against a wall, legs slightly apart, hands at your sides.

- Swing your injured arm forwards and upwards as high as you can manage.

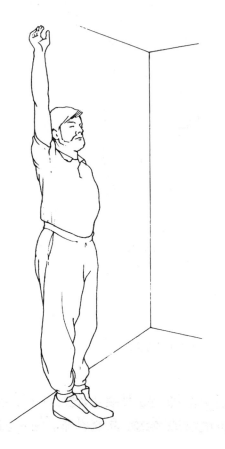

- Eventually you should be able to touch the wall above your head, but this will be difficult at first.

- Hold your arm up as high as you can for a second and then slowly lower.

- Repeat ten times.

34 SHOULDER RAISE

 To further strengthen the shoulder muscles.

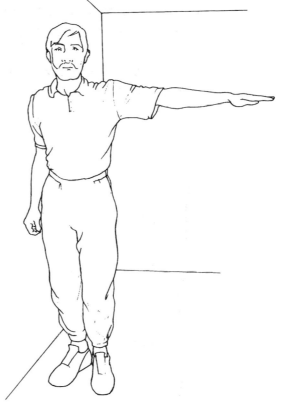

- Stand sideways next to a wall so that you have your good arm nearest the wall.

- Lean against the wall and lift the injured arm out sideways.

- Keep your elbow straight at all times.

- When you have moved your arm out as far as you can, hold this position for a second before lowering the arm.

- Repeat ten times.

 Aim to touch your ear with your arm.

 You can hold a small weight to do the exercise if you want, but practise without one first. A full coffee jar or baked-bean tin will do.

35 WINDMILL

 To generally loosen and warm down.

- Finish by gently 'windmilling' the shoulder.

- At first, keep your elbow bent so that your arm does not feel so heavy.

- Gradually, as you get stronger, let your arm straighten. Additionally, you can use simple shrugging of the shoulders to further help the overall strengthening and suppleness of your shoulders.

Recovery Programme for the Neck

The neck is probably the most vulnerable part of the spine. It is unprotected by other structures and has to move a heavy head in many different directions accurately and often quickly. Great leverage forces are exerted, particularly at the base of the neck, so the muscles are prone to fatigue, especially when spinal posture is poor.

Many people will have experienced what is commonly called 'wry neck', where the muscles spasm strongly and twist the neck in a painful way. Even small movements cause acute, stabbing pain. The large shoulder muscle, the trapezius, is often affected, feeling sore, tight, and limiting shoulder movements. This is not usually a serious condition but reminds us how much we use the neck muscles in daily life.

 Any tingling, weakness or numbness experienced in the arms or hands after a neck strain or injury requires immediate attention and you should seek advice.

All of the exercises in this **Recovery Programme for the Neck** can be performed either sitting or standing. They should be done in conjunction with the shoulder exercises. None of them should be painful, although they may be slightly uncomfortable to start with. It is very important that, if you have a stiff and painful neck, you do not allow it to stiffen further.

We all have a tendency to hold ourselves rather rigidly if suffering from neck pain. However, the same often applies to those who have no pain but whose neck has lost suppleness simply from lack of use. These exercises will help to maintain and improve your mobility and help prevent injury. They could therefore play a valuable part in your daily exercise routine, as well as being useful for self-help in the event of a neck injury.

 Anyone who has had a stroke, suffers from high blood pressure, vertigo, or arthritis in the neck, should check with an osteopath or chartered physiotherapist before doing any neck exercises.

36 FORWARD NECK FLEX

 To increase the range of neck flexion.

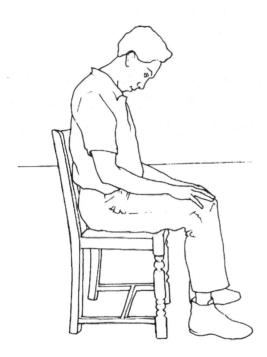

- Bend your head forwards gently and try to touch chin-to-chest.

- Lift your head backwards until it is just beyond the vertical.

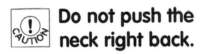 **Do not push the neck right back.**

- Repeat ten times.

37 SIDE NECK FLEX

 To increase the range of neck side-bending.

- Start with your head upright and bend it gently sideways towards one shoulder.

- Bring your head back up and continue in one movement to the other side.

- Perform five to ten repetitions.

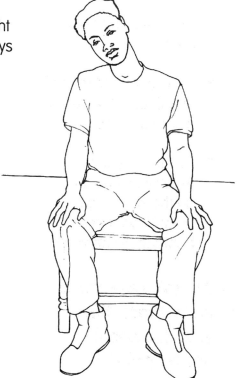

38 ROTATING NECK STRETCH

 To increase the range of neck rotation.

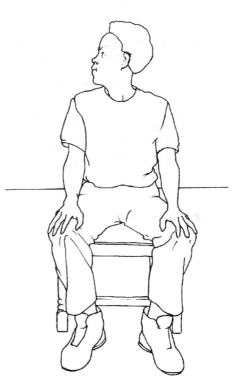

- Start with your head upright.

- Turn your head to the left and then to the right in a smooth action.

- Perform five to ten repetitions and then do the same again but with your head bent slightly forwards.

 Do not over-stretch. Remember, this exercise should not be painful.

Strengthening the neck with isometrics (muscle energy)

39 RESISTANCE EXERCISES

 To strengthen the muscles of the neck that provide support.

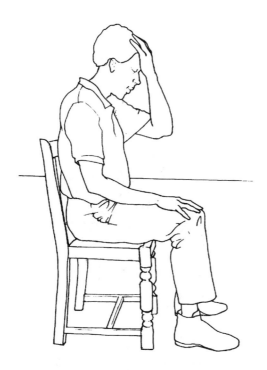

- Place one hand (preferably the side unaffected by your neck pain), against your forehead.

- Very gently press forward with your head into your hand for five seconds. Don't allow any actual movement to take place.

- Relax completely and then repeat three times.

 If it hurts, you are doing it too hard.

This same exercise can be variously repeated with the hand on the side of the head to strengthen side-bending or rotation, or on the back of the head. Please refer to the illustrations opposite.

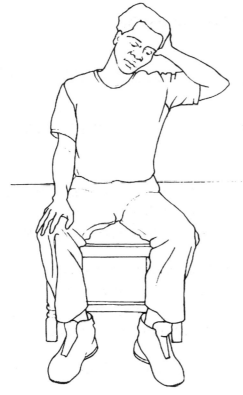

Exercise 39 repeated with the hand on the back of the head

Exercise 39 repeated with the hand on the side of the head

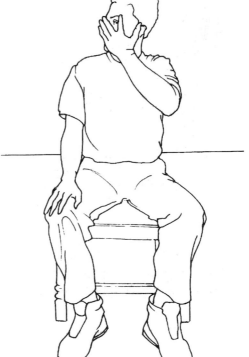

Exercise guide for recovery programmes

Recovery will mean different things to different individuals. Some people are quite content to recover to a point that allows them to comfortably perform their work and leisure activities. This may even be somewhat less than before they suffered an injury. Other people want one hundred per cent recovery; still others to be better than they were before they hurt themselves.

Exercise is meant to be beneficial. It is fruitless to continue performing any exercise (whether part of a programme or a specific exercise) if you experience pain. Some of you may still have aches and pains from your injury, and so it is important that you know when to stop.

- If you have any doubts, ask the advice of your GP, osteopath or physiotherapist.

- Any pain that is sharp enough at the time to make you jerk or to contract a limb sharply, or which initiates spasms, should be stopped.

- Any exercise that continues to cause pain and aching *after* you have completed your exercises should make you pause and check that you have chosen appropriate exercises, and that your technique is correct.

- As we all have different tolerance to pain and discomfort, use this principle as a rule of thumb: if your activity is painful, then stop. A sensation of *uncomfortable* stretch is acceptable, provided it *ceases* when you finish the exercise or stretch.

NB: The exercises that I have selected in the chart opposite are those that I feel are **most important in general terms**. However, this does not mean that you should use these exclusively. Please perform the others also to give yourself the best chance of full recovery.

Target Area	Stretch name and number	Page number	How long & how many	Duration
Back: Week One	Pre-exercise relaxation (17)	75	2 mins.	6 x per week
	Prone Extension A (18)	76	10 x	6 x per week
	Prone Extension B (19)	77	10 x	3 x per week
	Knee-to-chest A (20)	78	20 x	6 x per week
	Stomach Curl (22)	80	10 x	6 x per week
Back: Week Two	Pre-exercise relaxation (24)	82	2 mins.	6 x per week
	Prone Extension A (25)	83	10 x	6 x per week
	Prone Extension C (26)	84	10 x	3 x per week
	Knee-to-chest B (27) – Part 1	85	6 x	6 x per week
	– Part 2	86	20 x	6 x per week
	Stomach Curl (29)	88	10 x	6 x per week
Shoulders	Shoulder Rotation (31)	92	20 x each direction	6 x per week
	Wall-walking (32)	93	10 x	6 x per week
	Shoulder Swing (33)	94	10 x	6 x per week
	Towel Stretch (15)	54	15 secs. x 5	3 x per week
Neck	Forward Neck Flex (36)	99	10 x	6 x per week
	Side Neck Flex (37)	100	5–10 x	6 x per week
	Rotating Neck Stretch (38)	101	5–10 x	6 x per week

Legal Requirements

Rules on patient handling

Regulations came into operation on 1 January 1993 that relate to the responsibilities of employers for the safety of their staff. While these regulations and the guidance notes cannot be compulsorily applied to those who are caring for a relative, they do make good sense and should be read by all those who are carers.

The Regulations are made under the *Health and Safety at Work Act, 1974* and implement European Directive 90/269/EEC (*Manual Handling; Guidance on Regulations, 1992*) on 'the manual handling of loads', supplementing and in some cases superseding existing regulations and legal provisions.

The Health and Safety Executive note that over 25% of accidents reported to the enforcing authorities are associated with manual handling; they define manual handling as the 'transporting or supporting of loads by hand or by bodily force'. They comment that the great majority of injuries of a sprain or strain-type involve the back.

Employers' duties
All employers have a general duty to take all reasonable practical steps to ensure that their employees are safe and that their welfare is properly considered. Those who employ staff as carers also have a duty to those who are affected by their employees, such as patients and their relatives.

Employees who are contract staff can expect the same rights as those directly employed, under the *Health and Safety at Work Act, 1974.*

An employer is expected to assess risk of injury in 'manual handling', reduce these risks as far as is reasonably possible, and keep these assessments up to date. You, if you are an employee, can expect a written health and safety policy from your employer, who should make its procedures clear to you.

Employees' duties

All employees are also bound by provisions in the Act. They are expected to take reasonable care of their own safety and that of their colleagues when handling patients. You have a duty to co-operate with your employer, and this may include using properly any equipment provided by them.

Duties of the self-employed

Self-employed staff have the same responsibilities and duties to the people for whom they are working as do employed staff. However, the employer should determine what level of training and skill any self-employed staff possess before they start work, and give appropriate training if necessary.

Injuries at work

Responsibility of the employer

Employers are required to report all injuries that are major or fatal, require hospital admission for more than 24 hours, or lead to more than three days away from work (*The Reporting of Injuries, Diseases and Dangerous Occurrences Regulations, 1985*).

Employers should also make an accident book available to all employees at any reasonable time (*Regulation 25, Social Security (Claims and Payments) Regulations 1975*).

Employers are obliged to keep the accident book for three years from the date of its last entry.

Responsibility of the employee

It is most important that you as the employee report all accidents, however small. If there are later repercussions, then some record will have been kept. You are required by Social Security law to report any accidents as soon as possible.

Further Reading

Anderson, Bob (1981):
Stretching: Exercises for everyday fitness and for twenty-five individual sports,
Pelham Books.
ISBN 0 7207 1351 X

Cailliet, Rene, MD (1982, Third Edition):
Low Back Pain Syndrome,
FA Davis Company, Philadelphia.
ISBN 0 8036 1605 8

Grisogono, Vivian (1984):
Sports Injuries: A Self-Help Guide,
John Murray (Publishers) Ltd.
ISBN 0 7195 4111 5

Health and Safety Commission (1992):
Guidance on Manual Handling of Loads in the Health Services.
ISBN 0 11 886354 1

Health and Safety Commission (1992):
Manual Handling: Guidance on Regulations.
ISBN 0 11 886335 5

Hodgkinson, Liz (1988):
The Alexander Technique,
Judy Piatkus (Publishers) Ltd.
ISBN 0 86188 709 3

McKenzie, Robin (1985):
Treat Your Own Back,
Spinal Publications, New Zealand Ltd.
ISBN 0 9597746 6 1

National Back Pain Association (1992):
The Guide to the Handling of Patients,
National Back Pain Association, Middlesex.
ISBN 0 9507726 5 8

National Back Pain Association (1993):
A Carer's Guide to Moving and Handling Patients,
National Back Pain Association.
ISBN 0 9507726 7 4

National Back Pain Association (1991):
Lifting and Handling: An Ergonomic Approach,
National Back Pain Association.
ISBN 0 9507726 4 X

Pinckney, Callan (1990):
Callanetics for Your Back,
Guild Publishing. CN 1126

Sources of Further Information

Complementary therapies

Acupuncture
The Council for Acupuncture,
179 Gloucester Place, London, NW1 6DX.
Tel: 0171-724 5756.

Alexander Technique
The Society of Teachers of the Alexander Technique,
10, London House,
266, Fulham Road, London, SW10 9EL.
Tel: 0171-351 0828.

Osteopathy
Osteopathic Information Service,
PO Box 2074, Reading, Berkshire, RG1 4YR.
Tel: 01734 512051. Fax: 01734 566246.

The London School of Osteopathy
8, Lanark Square, Docklands, London, E14 9RE.
Tel: 0171-538 8334

National Organisations

Arthritis and Rheumatism Council
Copeman House,
St. Mary's Court, St. Mary's Gate, Chesterfield,
Derbyshire, S41 7TD.
Tel: 01246 558033.

Carers National Association
20-25 Glasshouse Yard, London, EC1A 4JS.
Tel: 0171-490 8818. Fax: 0171-490 8824.

Carers' Line: Tel: 0171-490 8898.

National Back Pain Association
31-33 Park Road, Teddington, Middlesex, TW11 0AB.
Tel: 0181-977 5474. Fax: 0181-943 5318.

Physiotherapy

Chartered Society of Physiotherapy
14 Bedford Row, London, WC1R 4ED.
Tel: 0171-242 1941. Fax: 0171-831 4509.

Index

Other titles from Pavilion Publishing

Pavilion publish a range of titles for staff, carers and users of caring services. A selection of our titles is listed below.

New Lifestyles for People With Learning Difficulties
Quality of care training workshops for staff based on the principle of normalisation.

New Lifestyles for People Who Use Mental Health Services
Quality of care training workshops for staff and service users based on the principle of normalisation.

Carers Need to Know
Essential information and training for GPs and primary health care teams.

New Lifestyles for Carers
A quality of care training workshop for staff and carers based on the principle of normalisation.

Working with Older People: 10 Training Workshops
A series of half-day workshop sessions designed to provide induction training in key areas or as a basis for refresher courses and in-house staff development.

Parenting Skills
A video training pack. Designed for use in running group courses on child management for parents, with the emphasis on normal everyday child behaviour.

For more information or a full catalogue of our products, please telephone 01273 623222.